Air Fryer Unmissable Recipes

A Collection of Delicious Air Fryer Recipes for
Your Daily Meals

Kira Hamm

TABLE OF CONTENT

this book has been derived from various sources. Please consult a licensed professional before attempting any techniques outlined in this book.

By reading this document, the reader agrees that under no circumstances is the author responsible for any losses, direct or indirect, which are incurred as a result of the use of information contained within this document, including, but not limited to, — errors, omissions, or inaccuracies.

Fried Scallops with Saffron Cream Sauce

Preparation Time:5 Minutes

Cooking Time: 2 minutes

Servings: 4

Ingredients:

- Olive oil for greasing
- 24 scallops, cleaned
- 2/3 cup heavy cream
- tbsp freshly squeezed lemon juice
- ¼ tsp dried crushed saffron threads

Directions:

1. Insert the dripping pan in the bottom part of the air fryer and preheat the oven at Air Fry mode 400 F for 2 to 3 minutes.
2. Lightly brush the rotisserie basket with some olive oil and fill with the scallops.
3. Close and fit the basket in the oven using the rotisserie lift and set the Timer for 2 minutes or until the scallops are golden brown on the outside.

4. Meanwhile, in a medium bowl, quickly whisk the heavy cream lemon juice and saffron threads.
5. When the scallops are ready, transfer to a serving plate and drizzle the sauce on top.
6. Enjoy immediately.

Nutrition: Calories 77 Total Fat 7.73g Total Carbs 1.05g Fiber 0g Protein 1.15g Sugar 0.66g Sodium 31mg

Easy Crab Cakes

Preparation Time: 10 minutes

Cooking Time: 10 minutes

Servings: 4

Ingredients:

- oz lump crab
- medium red bell pepper, deseeded and diced
- scallions, finely chopped
- tbsp mayonnaise
- tbsp panko bread crumbs
- 1 tbsp Dijon mustard
- 1 tsp old bay seasoning
- Olive oil for spraying
- lemon wedges for serving

Directions:

1. Insert the dripping pan in the bottom part of the air fryer and preheat the oven at Bake mode at 370 F for 2 to 3 minutes.
2. Meanwhile, in a medium bowl, mix all the ingredients except for the olive oil and lemon wedges until evenly distributed. From 4 to 6 firm patties from the mixture,

arrange on the cooking tray, and grease lightly with some olive oil. You may do this in two batches.

3. Fit the cooking tray on the middle rack and close the oven. Set the Timer to 10 minutes and cook until the Timer reads to the end, and the crab cakes are golden brown and well compacted.

4. Remove the crab cakes from the oven and serve with the lemon wedges.

Nutrition: Calories 246 Total Fat 6.19g Total Carbs 13.65g Fiber 1.5g Protein 33.16g Sugar 3.65g Sodium 338mg

Sweet Asian Style Salmon

Preparation Time:10 Minutes

Cooking Time: 12 minutes

Servings: 4

Ingredients:

- garlic cloves, minced
- tbsp fresh ginger paste
- tsp fresh orange zest
- ½ cup fresh orange juice
- ¼ cup of soy sauce
- tbsp plain vinegar
- 1 tbsp olive oil
- Salt to taste
- (5 oz) salmon fillets

Directions:

1. In a large bowl, mix all the ingredients except for the fish and place the fish in the sauce. Spoon the sauce well on top and cover the bowl with a plastic wrap. Allow marinating at room temperature for 30 minutes.
2. After 30 minutes, insert the dripping pan in the bottom part of the air fryer and preheat

the oven at Bake mode at 400 F for 2 to 3 minutes.

3. Using tongs, remove the fish from the sauce, making sure to shake off some marinade of the fish and place the cooking tray. You can work in two batches.

4. Slide the tray onto the top rack of the oven, close the oven, and set the Timer for 12 minutes, flipping the fish after 6 minutes.

5. Once ready, transfer the fish to serving plates and serve warm with steamed greens.

Nutrition: Calories 132, Total Fat 7.39g Total Carbs 8.72g Fiber 0.5g Protein 7.2g Sugar 5.96g Sodium 257mg

Zesty Ranch Fish Fillets

Preparation Time: 10 Minutes

Cooking Time: 13 minutes

Servings: 4

Ingredients:

- ¾ cup finely crushed cornflakes or panko breadcrumbs
- tbsp dry ranch-style dressing mix
- tsp fresh lemon zest
- ½ tbsp olive oil
- eggs, beaten
- white fish fillets
- Lemon wedges to garnish

Directions:

1. Insert the dripping pan in the bottom part of the air fryer and preheat the oven at Air Fry mode at 400 F for 2 to 3 minutes.
2. Mix the cornflakes, dressing mix, lemon zest, and oil on a shallow plate and then pour the eggs on another.
3. Working in two batches, dip the fish into the egg
4. drip off excess egg

13

5. and coat well in the cornflake's mixture on both sides.
6. Place the fish on the cooking tray and fix the tray on the middle rack of the oven. Close the oven and set the Timer for 13 minutes, and cook until the fish is golden brown and the fish flaky within.
7. Transfer to a serving plate and serve with the lemon wedges.

Nutrition: Calories 409 Total Fat 23.84g Total Carbs 3.79g Fiber 0.5g Protein 42.55g Sugar 1.41g Sodium 322mg

Dill Fish Chops

Preparation Time:10 Minutes

Cooking Time: 11 Minutes

Servings: 4

Ingredients:

- (5 oz) cod fillets, cut into 2-inch cubes
- ½ cup tapioca starch
- eggs
- cup almond flour
- 1 ½ dried fish seasoning
- 1 ½ dried dill
- Salt and black pepper to taste
- ½ tsp mustard powder
- Olive oil for greasing

Directions:

1. Insert the dripping pan in the bottom part of the air fryer and preheat the oven at Air Fry mode at 390 F for 2 to 3 minutes.
2. Pour the tapioca starch on a shallow plate, beat the eggs in a medium bowl, and mix the almond flour, fish seasoning
3. dill, salt, black pepper, and mustard powder on another plate.

4. Lightly coat the fish cubes in the starch, then dip in the eggs, and coat generously in the mustard mixture until well coated on all sides.

5. Spray the coated fish with a little olive oil and put it in the rotisserie basket. Fit the basket in the oven using the rotisserie ling and close the oven. Set the Timer for 11 minutes and cook until the fish is golden brown on the outside.

6. Transfer the crusted fish onto serving plates and serve warm with your favorite sauce.

Nutrition: Calories 206 Total Fat 4.02g Total Carbs 18.18g Fiber 0.4g Protein 22.79g Sugar 1.31g Sodium 398mg

Easy Fish Sticks with Chili Ketchup Sauce

Preparation Time:10 Minutes

Cooking Time: 12 Minutes

Servings: 4

Ingredients:

- fish sticks, store-bought
- ½ cup tomato ketchup
- tbsp Sriracha sauce
- 1 tbsp chopped fresh parsley to garnish
- Sliced pickles for serving

Directions:

1. Insert the dripping pan in the bottom part of the air fryer and preheat the oven at Air Fry mode at 390 F for 2 to 3 minutes.

2. Arrange the fish sticks on the cooking tray and fit onto the middle rack of the oven. Close and set the Timer for 12 minutes and cook until the fish sticks are golden brown and crispy.

3. Meanwhile, in a small bowl, mix the tomato ketchup, Sriracha sauce, and parsley until well combined and set aside for serving.

17

4. When the fish is ready, transfer onto serving plates and serve warm with the sauce and pickles.

Nutrition: Calories 341 Total Fat 2.53g Total Carbs 1.13g Fiber 0.4g Protein 73.57g Sugar 0.69g Sodium 568m

Packet Lobster Tail

Preparation Time: 10 minutes

Cooking Time: 27 minutes

Servings: 2

Ingredients:

- (6-oz. lobster tails, halved
- tbsp. salted butter; melted.
- 1 tsp. dried parsley.
- ½ tsp. Old Bay seasoning
- Juice of ½ medium lemons

Directions:

1. Place the two halved tails on an aluminum foil. Drizzle with butter, Old Bay seasoning and lemon juice.
2. Seal the foil packets, completely covering tails. Place into the air fryer basket
3. Adjust the temperature to 375 Degrees F and set the Timer for 12 minutes. Once done, sprinkle with dried parsley and serve immediately.

Nutrition: Calories: 234 Total Fat: 19 g Saturated Fat: 0 g Cholesterol: 0 mg Sodium: 0 mg Total Carbs: 7 g Fiber: 1 g Sugar: 0 g Protein: 23 g

Shrimp and Green Beans

Preparation Time:10 minutes

Cooking Time: 20 minutes

Servings: 4

Ingredients:

- ½ lb. green beans; trimmed and halved
- 1 lb. shrimp; peeled and deveined
- ¼ cup ghee; melted
- tbsp. cilantro; chopped.
- Juice of 1 lime
- A pinch of salt and black pepper

Directions:

1. In a pan that fits your air fryer, mix all the Ingredients: toss, introduce in the fryer and cook at 360°F for 15 minutes shaking the fryer halfway. Divide into bowls and serve

Nutrition: Calories: 222 Total Fat: 8 g Saturated Fat: 0 g Cholesterol: 0 mg Sodium: 0 mg Total Carbs: 5 g Fiber: 3 g Sugar: 0 g Protein: 10 g

Crab Dip

Preparation Time: 8 minutes

Cooking Time: 18 minutes

Servings: 4

Ingredients:

- oz. full-fat cream cheese; softened.
- (6-oz. cans lump crabmeat
- ¼ cup chopped pickled jalapeños.
- ¼ cup full-fat sour cream.
- ¼ cup sliced green onion
- ½ cup shredded Cheddar cheese
- ¼ cup full-fat mayonnaise
- 1 tbsp. lemon juice
- ½ tsp. hot sauce

Directions:

1. Place all Ingredients into a 4-cup round baking dish and stir until fully combined. Place dish into the air fryer basket Adjust the temperature to 400 Degrees F and set the Timer for 8 minutes. Dip will be bubbling and hot when done. Serve warm.

Nutrition: Calories: 441 Total Fat: 38 g Saturated Fat: 0 g Cholesterol: 0 mg Sodium: 0 mg Total Carbs:

2 g Fiber: 6 g Sugar: 0 g Protein: 18 g

Sesame Shrimp

Preparation Time: 8 minutes

Cooking Time: 15 minutes

Servings: 4

Ingredients:

- 1 lb. shrimp; peeled and deveined
- 1 tbsp. olive oil
- 1 tbsp. sesame seeds, toasted
- ½ tsp. Italian seasoning
- A pinch of salt and black pepper

Directions:

1. Take a bowl and mix the shrimp with the rest of the ingredients and toss well Put the shrimp in the air fryer's basket, cook at 370°F for 12 minutes, and divide into bowls and serve,

Nutrition: Calories: 199 Total Fat: 11 g Saturated Fat: 0 g Cholesterol: 0 mg Sodium: 0 mg Total Carbs: 4 g Fiber: 2 g Sugar: 0 g Protein: 11 g

Salmon and Cauliflower Rice

Preparation Time: 10 minutes

Cooking Time: 30 minutes

Servings: 4

Ingredients:

- salmon fillets; boneless
- ½ cup chicken stock
- 1 cup cauliflower, riced
- 1 tbsp. butter; melted
- 1 tsp. turmeric powder
- Salt and black pepper to taste

Directions:

1. In a pan that fits your air fryer, mix the cauliflower rice with the other ingredients except the salmon and toss Arrange the salmon fillets over the cauliflower rice, put the pan in the fryer and cook at 360°F for 25 minutes, flipping the fish after 15 minutes Divide everything between plates and serve

Nutrition: Calories: 241 Total Fat: 12 g Saturated Fat: 0 g Cholesterol: 0 mg Sodium: 0 mg Total Carbs:

6 g Fiber: 2 g Sugar: 0 g Protein: 12 g

Tilapia and Salsa

Preparation Time: 10 minutes

Cooking Time: 20 minutes

Servings: 4

Ingredients:

- tilapia fillets; boneless
- oz. canned tomatoes; chopped.
- tbsp. green onions; chopped.
- tbsp. sweet red pepper; chopped.
- 1 tbsp. balsamic vinegar
- 1 tbsp. olive oil
- A pinch of salt and black pepper

Directions:

1. Arrange the tilapia on a baking sheet that fits the air fryer and season with salt and pepper.
2. In a bowl, combine all the other Ingredients: toss and spread over the fish Introduce the pan in the fryer and cook at 350°F for 15 minutes
3. Divide the mix between plates and serve.

Nutrition: Calories: 221 Total Fat: 12 g Saturated Fat: 0 g Cholesterol: 0 mg Sodium: 0 mg Total Carbs:

5 g Fiber: 2 g Sugar: 0 g Protein: 14 g

Garlic Tilapia

Preparation Time:10 minutes

Cooking Time: 25 minutes

Servings: 4

Ingredients:

- tilapia fillets; boneless
- 1 bunch kale; chopped.
- garlic cloves; minced
- tbsp. olive oil
- 1 tsp. fennel seeds
- ½ tsp. red pepper flakes, crushed
- Salt and black pepper to taste

Directions:

1. In a pan that fits the fryer, combine all the Ingredients: put the pan in the fryer and cook at 360°F for 20 minutes Divide everything between plates and serve.

Nutrition: Calories 116 Fat 10 g Carbs 1.1 g Protein 6 g Calories: 240 Total Fat: 12 g Saturated Fat: 0 g Cholesterol: 0 mg Sodium: 0 mg Total Carbs: 4 g Fiber: 2 g Sugar: 0 g Protein: 12 g

Trout and Mint

Preparation Time: 10 minutes

Cooking Time: 21 minutes

Servings: 4

Ingredients:

- 1 avocado, peeled, pitted and roughly chopped.
- rainbow trout
- 1/3 pine nuts
- 1 cup olive oil + 3 tbsp.
- 1 cup parsley; chopped.
- garlic cloves; minced
- ½ cup mint; chopped.
- Zest of 1 lemon
- Juice of 1 lemon
- A pinch of salt and black pepper

Directions:

1. Pat dries the trout, season with salt and pepper and rub with 3 tbsp. oil
2. Put the fish in your air fryer's basket and cook for 8 minutes on each side. Divide the fish between plates and drizzle half of the lemon juice all over in a blender, combine

the rest of the oil with the remaining lemon juice, parsley, garlic, mint, lemon zest, pine nuts and the avocado and pulse well. Spread this over the trout and serve.

Nutrition: Calories: 240 Total Fat: 12 g Saturated Fat: 0 g Cholesterol: 0 mg Sodium: 0 mg Total Carbs: 6 g Fiber: 4 g Sugar: 0 g Protein: 9 g

Salmon and Coconut Sauce

Preparation Time:25 minutes

Cooking Time: 10 minutes

Servings: 4

Ingredients:

- salmon fillets; boneless
- 1/3 cup heavy cream
- ¼ cup lime juice
- ½ cup coconut; shredded
- ¼ cup coconut cream
- 1 tsp. lime zest; grated
- A pinch of salt and black pepper

Directions:

1. Take a bowl and mix all the ingredients except the salmon and whisk.
2. Arrange the fish in a pan that fits your air fryer, drizzle the coconut sauce all over, put the pan in the machine and cook at 360°F for 20 minutes Divide between plates and serve

Nutrition: Calories: 227 Total Fat: 12 g Saturated Fat: 0 g Cholesterol: 0 mg Sodium: 0 mg Total Carbs: 4 g Fiber: 2 g Sugar: 0 g Protein: 9 g

Simple Salmon

Preparation Time:10 minutes

Cooking Time: 22 minutes

Servings: 2

Ingredients:

- (4-oz. salmon fillets, skin removed
- 1 medium lemon
- tbsp. unsalted butter; melted.
- ½ tsp. dried dill
- ½ tsp. garlic powder

Directions:

1. Place each fillet on a 5" × 5" square of aluminum foil. Drizzle with butter and sprinkle with garlic powder.
2. Zest half of the lemon and sprinkle zest over salmon. Slice other half of the lemon and lay two slices on each piece of salmon. Sprinkle dill over salmon Gather and fold foil at the top and sides to fully close packets. Place foil packets into the air fryer basket. Adjust the temperature to 400 Degrees F and set the Timer for 12 minutes Salmon will be easily flaked and have an

internal temperature of at least 145 Degrees F when fully cooked.

Nutrition: Calories: 252 Total Fat: 15 g Saturated Fat: 0 g Cholesterol: 0 mg Sodium: 0 mg Total Carbs: 2 g Fiber: 4 g Sugar: 0 g Protein: 29 g

Cajun Salmon

Preparation Time: 5 minutes

Cooking Time: 12 minutes

Servings: 2

Ingredients:

- (4-oz. salmon fillets, skin removed
- tbsp. unsalted butter; melted.
- 1 tsp. paprika
- ¼ tsp. ground black pepper
- 1/8 Tsp. ground cayenne pepper
- ½ tsp. garlic powder

Directions:

1. Brush each fillet with butter. Combine remaining ingredients in a small bowl and then rub onto fish. Place fillets into the air fryer basket Adjust the temperature to 390 Degrees F and set the Timer for 7 minutes. When fully cooked, internal temperature will be 145 Degrees F. Serve immediately.

Nutrition: Calories: 253 Total Fat: 16 g Saturated Fat: 0 g Cholesterol: 0 mg Sodium: 0 mg Total Carbs: 4 g Fiber: 4 g Sugar: 0 g Protein: 29 g

Salmon and Sauce

Preparation Time:10 minutes

Cooking Time: 25 minutes

Servings: 4

Ingredients:

- salmon fillets; boneless
- garlic cloves; minced
- ¼ cup ghee; melted
- ½ cup heavy cream
- 1 tbsp. chives; chopped.
- 1 tsp. lemon juice
- 1 tsp. dill; chopped.
- A pinch of salt and black pepper

Directions:

1. Take a bowl and mix all the ingredients except the salmon and whisk well.
2. Arrange the salmon in a pan that fits the air fryer, drizzle the sauce all over, introduce the pan in the machine and cook at 360°F for 20 minutes. Divide everything between plates and serve

Nutrition: Calories: 220 Total Fat: 14 g Saturated Fat: 0 g Cholesterol: 0 mg Sodium: 0 mg Total Carbs:

5 g Fiber: 2 g Sugar: 0 g Protein: 12 g

Parmesan Cod

Preparation Time: 10 minutes

Cooking Time: 20 minutes

Servings: 4

Ingredients:

- cod fillets; boneless
- A drizzle of olive oil
- spring onions; chopped.
- 1 cup parmesan
- tbsp. balsamic vinegar
- Salt and black pepper to taste

Directions:

1. Season fish with salt, pepper, grease with the oil and coat it in parmesan.
2. Put the fillets in your air fryer's basket and cook at 370°F for 14 minutes. Meanwhile, in a bowl, mix the spring onions with salt, pepper and the vinegar and whisk Divide the cod between plates, drizzle the spring onions mix all over and serve with a side salad

Nutrition: Calories: 220 Total Fat: 12 g Saturated Fat: 0 g Cholesterol: 0 mg Sodium: 0 mg Total Carbs:

5 g Fiber: 2 g Sugar: 0 g Protein: 13 g

Cod and Endives

Preparation Time: 10 minutes

Cooking Time: 25 minutes

Servings: 4

Ingredients:

- salmon fillets; boneless
- endives; shredded
- tbsp. olive oil
- ½ tsp. sweet paprika
- Salt and black pepper to the taste

Directions:

1. In a pan that fits the air fryer, combine the fish with the rest of the Ingredients: toss, introduce in the fryer and cook at 350°F for 20 minutes, flipping the fish halfway Divide between plates and serve right away

Nutrition: Calories: 243Total Fat: 13 g Saturated Fat: 0 g Cholesterol: 0 mg Sodium: 0 mg Total Carbs: 6 g Fiber: 3 g Sugar: 0 g Protein: 14 g

Cod and Tomatoes

Preparation Time:10 minutes

Cooking Time: 20 minutes

Servings: 4

Ingredients:

- 1 cup cherry tomatoes; halved
- cod fillets, skinless and boneless
- tbsp. olive oil
- tbsp. cilantro; chopped.
- Salt and black pepper to taste

Directions:

1. In a baking dish that fits your air fryer, mix all the Ingredients: toss gently.
2. Introduce in your air fryer and cook at 370°F for 15 minutes
3. Divide everything between plates and serve right away.

Nutrition: Calories: 248 Total Fat: 11 g Saturated Fat: 0 g Cholesterol: 0 mg Sodium: 0 mg Total Carbs: 5 g Fiber: 2 g Sugar: 0 g Protein: 11 g

Salmon Burgers

Preparation Time:10 minutes

Cooking Time: 10 minutes

Servings: 4

Ingredients:

- oz. can salmon, drain & flake
- ¼ cup onion, chopped fine
- 1 egg
- ¼ cup multi-grain crackers, crushed
- tsp fresh dill, chopped
- ¼ tsp pepper
- Nonstick cooking spray

Directions:

1. In a medium bowl, combine all ingredients until combined. Form into 4 patties.

2. Lightly spray fryer basket with cooking spray. Place the baking pan in position 2 of the oven.

3. Set oven to air fryer on 350°F.

4. Place the patties in the basket and set on baking pan. Set Timer for 8 minutes. Cook until burgers are golden brown, turning

over halfway through cooking Time. Serve on toasted buns with choice of toppings.

Nutrition: Calories: 330 Total Fat: 10 g Saturated Fat: 2 g Cholesterol: 0 mg Sodium: 643 mg Total Carbs: 11 g Fiber: 0 g Sugar: 0 g Protein: 24 g

Air Fried Haddock Filets

Preparation Time: 10 minutes

Cooking Time: 20 minutes

Servings: 8

Ingredients:

- Nonstick cooking spray
- egg whites
- ½ tsp dill
- ½ tsp pepper
- 1 cup cornflakes, crushed
- lbs. haddock fillets, cut in 8 pieces

Directions:

1. Place baking pan in position 2 of the oven. Lightly spray fryer basket with cooking spray.
2. In a shallow bowl, whisk together egg whites, dill, and pepper.
3. Place crushed cornflakes in a separate shallow dish.
4. Dip fish in egg mixture, then cornflakes, coating completely. Place in fryer basket.
5. Place basket on the baking pan and set oven to air fryer on 400°F. Cook 18-20

minutes, turning over halfway through, until fish flakes easily with a fork. Serve.

Nutrition: Calories: 193 Total Fat: 1 g Saturated Fat: 0 g Cholesterol: 0 mg Sodium: 568 mg Total Carbs: 7 g Fiber: 0 g Sugar: 1 g Protein: 39 g

Crispy Coated Scallops

Preparation Time:10 minutes

Cooking Time: 10 minutes

Servings: 4

Ingredients:

- Nonstick cooking spray
- 1 lb. sea scallops, patted dry
- 1 teaspoon onion powder
- ½ tsp pepper
- 1 egg
- 1 tbsp. water
- ¼ cup Italian breadcrumbs
- Paprika
- 1 tbsp. fresh lemon juice

Directions:

1. Lightly spray fryer basket with cooking spray. Place baking pan in position 2 of the oven.
2. Sprinkle scallops with onion powder and pepper.
3. In a shallow dish, whisk together egg and water.

4. Place bread crumbs in a separate shallow dish.

5. Dip scallops in egg then bread crumbs coating them lightly. Place in fryer basket and lightly spray with cooking spray. Sprinkle with paprika.

6. Place the basket on the baking pan and set oven to air fryer on 400°F. Bake 10-12 minutes until scallops are firm on the inside and golden brown on the outside. Drizzle with lemon juice and serve.

Nutrition: Calories: 122 Total Fat: 2 g Saturated Fat: 1 g Cholesterol: 0 mg Sodium: 563 mg Total Carbs: 10 g Fiber: 1 g Sugar: 1 g Protein: 0 g

Tasty Tuna Loaf

Preparation Time:10 minutes

Cooking Time: 40 minutes

Servings: 6

Ingredients:

- Nonstick cooking spray
- oz. can chunk white tuna in water, drain & flake
- ¾ cup bread crumbs
- 1 onion, chopped fine
- eggs, beaten
- ¼ cup milk
- ½ tsp fresh lemon juice
- ½ tsp dill
- 1 tbsp. fresh parsley, chopped
- ½ tsp salt
- ½ tsp pepper

Directions:

1. Place rack in position 1 of the oven. Spray a 9-inch loaf pan with cooking spray.
2. In a large bowl, combine all ingredients until thoroughly mixed. Spread evenly in pan.

3. Set oven to bake on 350°F for 45 minutes. After 5 minutes, place the pan in the oven and cook 40 minutes, or until top is golden brown. Slice and serve.

Nutrition: Calories: 169 Total Fat: 5 g Saturated Fat: 1 g Cholesterol: 0 mg Sodium: 540 mg Total Carbs: 13 g Fiber: 1 g Sugar: 3 g Protein: 18 g

Maryland Crab Cakes

Preparation Time:10 minutes

Cooking Time: 10 minutes

Servings: 6

Ingredients:

- Nonstick cooking spray
- eggs
- 1 cup Panko breadcrumbs
- 1 stalk celery, chopped
- tbsp. mayonnaise
- 1 tsp Worcestershire sauce
- ¼ cup mozzarella cheese, grated
- 1 tsp Italian seasoning
- 1 tbsp. fresh parsley, chopped
- 1 tsp pepper
- ¾ lb. Lump crabmeat, drained

Directions:

1. Place baking pan in position 2 of the oven. Lightly spray the fryer basket with cooking spray.
2. In a large bowl, combine all ingredients except crab meat, mix well.

3. Fold in crab carefully so it retains some chunks. Form mixture into 12 patties.

4. Place patties in a single layer in the fryer basket. Place the basket on the baking pan.

5. Set oven to air fryer on 350°F for 10 minutes. Cook until golden brown, turning over halfway through cooking Time. Serve immediately.

Nutrition: Calories: 172 Total Fat: 8 g Saturated Fat: 2 g Cholesterol: 0 mg Sodium: 527 mg Total Carbs: 14 g Fiber: 1 g Sugar: 1 g Protein: 16 g

Mediterranean Sole

Preparation Time:15 minutes

Cooking Time: 20 minutes

Servings: 6

Ingredients:

- Nonstick cooking spray
- tbsp. olive oil
- scallions, sliced thin
- cloves garlic, diced fine
- tomatoes, chopped
- ½ cup dry white wine
- tbsp. fresh parsley, chopped fine
- 1 tsp oregano
- 1 tsp pepper
- lbs. sole, cut in 6 pieces
- oz. feta cheese, crumbled

Directions:

1. Place the rack in position 1 of the oven. Spray an 8x11-inch baking dish with cooking spray.
2. Heat the oil in a medium skillet over medium heat. Add scallions and garlic and cook until tender, stirring frequently.

3. Add the tomatoes, wine, parsley, oregano, and pepper. Stir to mix. Simmer for 5 minutes, or until sauce thickens. Remove from heat.
4. Pour half the sauce on the bottom of the dish. Lay fish on top then pour remaining sauce over the top. Sprinkle with feta.
5. Set the oven to bake on 400°F for 25 minutes. After 5 minutes, place the baking dish on the rack and cook 15-18 minutes or until fish flakes easily with a fork. Serve immediately.

Nutrition: Calories: 220 Total Fat: 12 g Saturated Fat: 4 g Cholesterol: 0 mg Sodium: 631 mg Total Carbs: 6 g Fiber: 2 g Sugar: 4 g Protein: 22 g

Spicy Grilled Halibut

Preparation Time: 30 minutes

Cooking Time: 10 minutes

Servings: 4

Ingredients:

- ½ cup fresh lemon juice
- jalapeno peppers, seeded & chopped fine
- 6 oz. halibut fillets
- Nonstick cooking spray
- ¼ cup cilantro, chopped

Directions:

1. In a small bowl, combine lemon juice and chilies, mix well.
2. Place fish in a large Ziploc bag and add marinade. Toss to coat. Refrigerate 30 minutes.
3. Lightly spray the baking pan with cooking spray. Set oven to broil on 400°F for 15 minutes.
4. After 5 minutes, lay fish on the pan and place in position 2 of the oven. Cook 10 minutes, or until fish flakes easily with a

fork. Turn fish over and brush with marinade halfway through cooking Time.

5. Sprinkle with cilantro before serving.

Nutrition: Calories: 328 Total Fat: 24 g Saturated Fat: 4 g Cholesterol: 0 mg Sodium: 137 mg Total Carbs: 3 g Fiber: 0 g Sugar: 1 g Protein: 25 g

Tropical Shrimp Skewers

Preparation Time:15 minutes

Cooking Time: 5 minutes

Servings: 4

Ingredients:

- 1 tbsp. lime juice
- 1 tbsp. honey
- ¼ tsp red pepper flakes
- ¼ tsp pepper
- ¼ tsp ginger
- Nonstick cooking spray
- 1 lb. medium shrimp, peel, devein & leave tails on
- cups peaches drain & chop
- ½ green bell pepper, chopped fine
- ¼ cup scallions, chopped

Directions:

1. Soak 8 small wooden skewers in water for 15 minutes.
2. In a small bowl, whisk together lime juice, honey and spices Transfer 2 tablespoons of the mixture to a medium bowl.

3. Place the baking pan in position 2 of the oven. Lightly spray fryer basket with cooking spray. Set oven to broil on 400°F for 10 minutes.

4. Thread 5 shrimp on each skewer and brush both sides with marinade. Place in basket and after 5 minutes, place on the baking pan. Cook 4-5 minutes or until shrimp turn pink.

5. Add peaches, bell pepper, and scallions to reserved honey mixture, mix well. Divide salsa evenly between serving plates and top with 2 skewers each. Serve immediately.

Nutrition: Calories: 181 Total Fat: 1 g Saturated Fat: 0 g Cholesterol: 0 mg Sodium: 650 mg Total Carbs: 27 g Fiber: 2 g Sugar: 21 g Protein: 16 g

Seafood Mac n Cheese

Preparation Time:20 minutes

Cooking Time: 30 minutes

Servings: 8

Ingredients:

- Nonstick cooking spray
- 16 oz. macaroni
- tbsp. butter, divided
- ¾ lb. medium shrimp, peel, devein, & cut in ½-inch pieces
- ½ cup Italian panko bread crumbs
- 1 cup onion, chopped fine
- 1 ½ tsp garlic, diced fine
- 1/3 cup flour
- cups milk
- 1/8 tsp nutmeg
- ½ tsp Old Bay seasoning
- 1 tsp salt
- ¾ tsp pepper
- 1 1/3 cup Parmesan cheese, grated
- 1 1/3 cup Swiss cheese, grated
- 1 1/3 cup sharp cheddar cheese, grated
- ½ lb. lump crab meat, cooked

Directions:

1. Place wire rack in position 1 of the oven. Spray a 7x11-inch baking dish with cooking spray.
2. Cook macaroni according to package Directions: shortening cooking Time by 2 minutes. Drain and rinse with cold water.
3. Melt 1 tablespoon butter in a large skillet over med-high heat. Add shrimp and cook, stirring
4. until they turn pink. Remove from heat.
5. Melt remaining butter in a large saucepan over medium heat. Once melted, transfer 2 tablespoons to a small bowl and mix in bread crumbs.
6. Add onions and garlic to saucepan and cook, stirring
7. until they soften.
8. Whisk in flour and cook 1 minute, until smooth.
9. Whisk in milk until there are no lumps. Bring to a boil, reduce heat and simmer until thickened, whisking constantly.

10. Whisk in seasonings. Stir in cheese until melted and smooth. Fold in macaroni and seafood. Transfer to dish. Sprinkle bread crumb mixture evenly over top.

11. Set oven to bake on 400°F for 25 minutes. After 5 minutes, place dish on the rack and bake 20 minutes, until topping is golden brown and sauce is bubbly. Let cool 5 minutes before serving.

Nutrition: Calories: 672 Total Fat: 26 g Saturated Fat: 15 g Cholesterol: 0 mg Sodium: 0 mg Total Carbs: 68 g Fiber: 7 g Sugar: 7 g Protein: 39 g

Crispy Air Fried Sushi Roll

Preparation Time: 5 minutes

Cooking Time: 15 minutes

Servings: 12

Ingredients:

- Kale Salad:
- 1 tbsp. sesame seeds
- ¾ tsp. soy sauce
- ¼ tsp. ginger
- 1/8 tsp. garlic powder
- ¾ tsp. toasted sesame oil
- ½ tsp. rice vinegar
- 1 ½ C. chopped kale
- Sushi Rolls:
- ½ of a sliced avocado
- sheets of sushi nori
- 1 batch cauliflower rice
- Sriracha Mayo:
- Sriracha sauce
- ¼ C. vegan mayo
- Coating:
- ½ C. panko breadcrumbs

Directions:

1. Combine all of kale salad ingredients together, tossing well. Set to the side.
2. Lay out a sheet of nori and spread a handful of rice on. Then place 2-3 tbsp. of kale salad over rice, followed by avocado. Roll up sushi.
3. To make mayo, whisk mayo ingredients together until smooth.
4. Add breadcrumbs to a bowl. Coat sushi rolls in crumbs till coated and add to air fryer.
5. Cook rolls 10 minutes at 390 degrees, shaking gently at 5 minutes.
6. Slice each roll into 6-8 pieces and enjoy!

Nutrition: Calories: 267 Total Fat: 13 g Saturated Fat: 0 g Cholesterol: 0 mg Sodium: 0 mg Total Carbs: 0 g Fiber: 0 g Sugar: 3 g Protein: 6 g

Honey Glazed Salmon

Preparation Time: 5 minutes

Cooking Time: 5 minutes

Servings: 2

Ingredients:

- 1 tsp. water
- tsp. rice wine vinegar
- tbsp. low-sodium soy sauce
- tbsp. raw honey
- salmon fillets

Directions:

1. Combine water, vinegar, honey, and soy sauce together. Pour half of this mixture into a bowl.

2. Place salmon in one bowl of marinade and let chill 2 hours.

3. Ensure your air fryer is preheated to 356 degrees and add salmon.

4. Cook 8 minutes, flipping halfway through. Baste salmon with some of the remaining marinade mixture and cook another 5 minutes.

5. To make a sauce to serve salmon with, pour remaining marinade mixture into a saucepan, heating till simmering. Let simmer 2 minutes. Serve drizzled over salmon!

Nutrition: Calories: 390 Total Fat: 8 g Saturated Fat: 0 g Cholesterol: 0 mg Sodium: 0 mg Total Carbs: 0 g Fiber: 0 g Sugar: 5 g Protein: 16 g

Parmesan Shrimp

Preparation Time:5 minutes

Cooking Time: 10 minutes

Servings: 4 - 6

Ingredients:

- tbsp. olive oil
- 1 tsp. onion powder
- 1 tsp. basil
- ½ tsp. oregano
- 1 tsp. pepper
- 2/3 C. grated parmesan cheese
- minced garlic cloves
- pounds of jumbo cooked shrimp (peeled/deveined)

Directions:

1. Mix all seasonings together and gently toss shrimp with mixture.
2. Spray olive oil into air fryer basket and add seasoned shrimp.
3. Cook 8-10 minutes at 350 degrees.
4. Squeeze lemon juice over shrimp right before devouring!

Nutrition: Calories: 351 Total Fat: 11 g Saturated

Fat: 0 g Cholesterol: 0 mg Sodium: 0 mg Total Carbs: 0 g Fiber: 0 g Sugar: 1 g Protein: 19 g

Bacon Wrapped Scallops

Preparation Time:5 minutes

Cooking Time: 10 minutes

Servings: 4

Ingredients:

- 1 tsp. paprika
- 1 tsp. lemon pepper
- slices of center-cut bacon
- 20 raw sea scallops

Directions:

1. Rinse and drain scallops, placing on paper towels to soak up excess moisture.
2. Cut slices of bacon into 4 pieces.
3. Wrap each scallop with a piece of bacon, using toothpicks to secure. Sprinkle wrapped scallops with paprika and lemon pepper.
4. Spray air fryer basket with olive oil and add scallops.
5. Cook 5-6 minutes at 400 degrees, making sure to flip halfway through.

Nutrition: Calories: 389 Total Fat: 17 g Saturated Fat: 0 g Cholesterol: 0 mg Sodium: 0 mg Total Carbs:

0 g Fiber: 0 g Sugar: 1 g Protein: 210 g

Air Fryer Fish Tacos

Preparation Time:5 minutes

Cooking Time: 5 minutes

Servings: 4

Ingredients:

- 1 pound cod
- 1 tbsp. cumin
- ½ tbsp. chili powder
- 1 ½ C. almond flour
- 1 ½ C. coconut flour
- ounces Mexican beer
- eggs

Directions:

1. Whisk beer and eggs together.
2. Whisk flours, pepper, salt, cumin, and chili powder together.
3. Slice cod into large pieces and coat in egg mixture then flour mixture.
4. Spray bottom of your air fryer basket with olive oil and add coated codpieces.
5. Cook 15 minutes at 375 degrees.
6. Serve on lettuce leaves topped with homemade salsa!

Nutrition: Calories: 178 Total Fat: 10 g Saturated Fat: 0 g Cholesterol: 0 mg Sodium: 0 mg Total Carbs: 0 g Fiber: 0 g Sugar: 1 g Protein: 19 g

Salmon Croquettes

Preparation Time: 5 minutes

Cooking Time: 15 minutes

Servings: 6 - 8

Ingredients:

- Panko breadcrumbs
- Almond flour
- egg whites
- tbsp. chopped chives
- tbsp. minced garlic cloves
- ½ C. chopped onion
- 2/3 C. grated carrots
- 1-pound chopped salmon fillet

Directions:

1. Mix together all Ingredients: minus breadcrumbs, flour, and egg whites.
2. Shape mixture into balls. Then coat them in flour, then egg
3. and then breadcrumbs. Drizzle with olive oil.
4. Add coated salmon balls to air fryer and cook 6 minutes at 350 degrees. Shake and

cook an additional 4 minutes until golden in color.

Nutrition: Calories: 503 Total Fat: 9 g Saturated Fat: 0 g Cholesterol: 0 mg Sodium: 0 mg Total Carbs: 61 g Fiber: 0 g Sugar: 4 g Protein: 5 g

Panko-Crusted Tilapia

Preparation Time: 5 minutes

Cooking Time: 5 minutes

Servings: 3

Ingredients:

- tsp. Italian seasoning
- tsp. lemon pepper
- 1/3 C. panko breadcrumbs
- 1/3 C. egg whites
- 1/3 C. almond flour
- tilapia fillets
- Olive oil

Directions:

1. Place panko, egg whites, and flour into separate bowls. Mix lemon pepper and Italian seasoning in with breadcrumbs.
2. Pat tilapia fillets dry. Dredge in flour, then egg
3. then breadcrumb mixture. Add to air fryer basket and spray lightly with olive oil.
4. Cook 10-11 minutes at 400 degrees, making sure to flip halfway through cooking.

Nutrition: Calories: 256 Total Fat: 9 g Saturated Fat: 0 g Cholesterol: 0 mg Sodium: 0 mg Total Carbs: 0 g Fiber: 0 g Sugar: 5 g Protein: 39 g

Friedamari

Preparation Time: 5 minutes

Cooking Time: 15 minutes

Servings: 6 - 8

Ingredients:

- ½ tsp. salt
- ½ tsp. Old Bay seasoning
- 1/3 C. plain cornmeal
- ½ C. semolina flour
- ½ C. almond flour
- 5-6 C. olive oil
- 1 ½ pounds baby squid

Directions:

1. Rinse squid in cold water and slice tentacles, keeping just ¼-inch of the hood in one piece.
2. Combine 1-2 pinches of pepper, salt, Old Bay seasoning
3. cornmeal, and both flours together. Dredge squid pieces into flour mixture and place into air fryer. Spray liberally with olive oil.
4. Cook 15 minutes at 345 degrees till coating turns a golden brown.

Nutrition: Calories: 211 Total Fat: 6 g Saturated Fat: 0 g Cholesterol: 0 mg Sodium: 0 mg Total Carbs: 0 g Fiber: 0 g Sugar: 1 g Protein: 21 g

Air Fryer Salmon Patties

Preparation Time: 5 minutes

Cooking Time: 15 minutes

Servings: 4

Ingredients:

- 1 tbsp. olive oil
- 1 tbsp. ghee
- ¼ tsp. salt
- 1/8 tsp. pepper
- 1 egg
- 1 C. almond flour
- 1 can wild Alaskan pink salmon

Directions:

1. Drain can of salmon into a bowl and keep liquid. Discard skin and bones.
2. Add salt, pepper, and egg to salmon, mixing well with hands to incorporate. Make patties.
3. Dredge in flour and remaining egg. If it seems dry, spoon reserved salmon liquid from the can onto patties.

4. Add patties to air fryer. Cook 7 minutes at 378 degrees till golden, making sure to flip once during cooking process.

Nutrition: Calories: 437 Total Fat: 12 g Saturated Fat: 0 g Cholesterol: 0 mg Sodium: 0 mg Total Carbs: 55 g Fiber: 0 g Sugar: 2 g Protein: 24 g

Louisiana Shrimp Po Boy

Preparation Time:10 minutes

Cooking Time: 15 minutes

Servings: 4

Ingredients:

- 1 tsp. creole seasoning
- slices of tomato
- Lettuce leaves
- ¼ C. buttermilk
- ½ C. Louisiana Fish Fry
- 1-pound deveined shrimp
- Remoulade sauce:
- 1 chopped green onion
- 1 tsp. hot sauce
- 1 tsp. Dijon mustard
- ½ tsp. creole seasoning
- 1 tsp. Worcestershire sauce
- Juice of ½ a lemon
- ½ C. vegan mayo

Directions:

1. To make the sauce, combine all sauce ingredients until well incorporated. Chill while you cook shrimp.

2. Mix seasonings together and liberally season shrimp.

3. Add buttermilk to a bowl. Dip each shrimp into milk and place in a Ziploc bag. Chill half an hour to marinate.

4. Add fish fry to a bowl. Take shrimp from marinating bag and dip into fish fry, then add to air fryer.

5. Ensure your air fryer is preheated to 400 degrees.

6. Spray shrimp with olive oil. Cook 5 minutes, flip and then cook another 5 minutes.

7. Assemble "Keto" Po Boy by adding sauce to lettuce leaves, along with shrimp and tomato.

Nutrition: Calories: 337 Total Fat: 12 g Saturated Fat: 0 g Cholesterol: 0 mg Sodium: 0 mg Total Carbs: 55 g Fiber: 0 g Sugar: 2 g Protein: 24 g

Bang Frieda Mari Panko Breaded Fried Shrimp

Preparation Time:5 minutes

Cooking Time: 15 minutes

Servings: 4

Ingredients:

- 1 tsp. paprika
- Montreal chicken seasoning
- ¾ C. panko bread crumbs
- ½ C. almond flour
- 1 egg white
- 1-pound raw shrimp (peeled and deveined)
- Bang Frieda Mari Sauce:
- ¼ C. sweet chili sauce
- tbsp. sriracha sauce
- 1/3 C. plain Greek yogurt

Directions:

1. Ensure your air fryer is preheated to 400 degrees.
2. Season all shrimp with seasonings.
3. Add flour to one bowl, egg white in another, and breadcrumbs to a third.

4. Dip seasoned shrimp in flour, then egg whites, and then breadcrumbs.
5. Spray coated shrimp with olive oil and add to air fryer basket.
6. Cook 4 minutes, flip, and cook an additional 4 minutes.
7. To make the sauce, mix together all sauce ingredients until smooth.

Nutrition: Calories: 212 Total Fat: 1 g Saturated Fat: 0 g Cholesterol: 0 mg Sodium: 0 mg Total Carbs: 12 g Fiber: 0 g Sugar: 0.5 g Protein: 37 g

3-Ingredient Air Fryer Catfish

Preparation Time:5 minutes

Cooking Time: 15 minutes

Servings: 4

Ingredients:

- 1 tbsp. chopped parsley
- 1 tbsp. olive oil
- ¼ C. seasoned fish fry
- catfish fillets

Directions:

1. Ensure your air fryer is preheated to 400 degrees.
2. Rinse off catfish fillets and pat dry.
3. Add fish fry seasoning to Ziploc baggie, then catfish. Shake bag and ensure fish gets well coated.
4. Spray each fillet with olive oil.
5. Add fillets to air fryer basket. Cook 10 minutes. Then flip and cook another 2-3 minutes.

Nutrition: Calories: 208 Total Fat: 5 g Saturated Fat: 0 g Cholesterol: 0 mg Sodium: 0 mg Total Carbs: 8

g Fiber: 0 g Sugar: 0.5 g Protein: 17 g

Healthy Fish and Chips

Preparation Time:5 minutes

Cooking Time: 15 minutes

Servings: 3

Ingredients:

- Old Bay seasoning
- ½ C. panko breadcrumbs
- 1 egg
- tbsp. almond flour
- 4–6-ounce tilapia fillets
- Frozen crinkle cut fries

Directions:

1. Add almond flour to one bowl, beat egg in another bowl, and add panko breadcrumbs to the third bowl, mixed with Old Bay seasoning.
2. Dredge tilapia in flour, then egg
3. and then breadcrumbs.
4. Place coated fish in air fryer along with fries.
5. Cook 15 minutes at 390 degrees.

Nutrition: Calories: 219 Total Fat: 5 g Saturated Fat: 0 g Cholesterol: 0 mg Sodium: 0 mg Total Carbs: 18

g Fiber: 0 g Sugar: 1 g Protein: 25 g

Fish in Parchment Paper

Preparation Time:10 minutes

Cooking Time: 25 minutes

Servings: 2

Ingredients:

- oz. cod fillets thawed
- 1 tbsp. Oil
- 1/2 cup julienned carrots
- sprigs tarragon
- 1/2 cup red peppers
- 1/2 tsp. Black Pepper
- pats melted butter
- 1 tbsp. lemon juice
- 1 tbsp. Salt divided
- 1/2 cup julienned fennel bulbs

Directions:

1. Take a bowl and add melted butter, tarragon, 1/2 tsp. salt, and lemon juice. Combine well until unless you get a creamy sauce. Put the julienned vegetable and stir well. Set it aside. Slice two squares of parchment big enough to hold the fish and vegetables. Spray the fish fillets with

cooking oil spray and apply salt & pepper to all sides of the fillets. Lay down one filet down on each parchment square. Top each fillet with half of the vegetables. Pour any leftover sauce over the vegetables. Fold over the parchment paper and crimp the sides to hold fish, veggies and sauce carefully inside the packet. Place the packets inside the air fryer toaster oven basket. Set your air fryer toaster oven to 350F for 15 minutes. Put each packet to a plate and open just before serving.

Nutrition: Calories: 251 Total Fat: 12 g Saturated Fat: 0 g Cholesterol: 0 mg Sodium: 0 mg Total Carbs: 8 g Fiber: 2 g Sugar: 0 g Protein: 26 g

Buttery Scallops

Preparation Time:10 minutes

Cooking Time: 25 minutes

Serving: 8

Ingredients:

- `2 lb. Scallops
- `6 tablespoons butter, melted
- `2 tablespoons dry white wine
- `1 tablespoon lemon juice
- `1/2 cup parmesan cheese, grated
- `1 teaspoon salt
- `1/2 teaspoon black pepper
- `1 teaspoon garlic powder
- `1 teaspoon dried parsley
- `1/8 teaspoon cayenne pepper
- `1/4 teaspoon sweet paprika
- `2 tablespoons parsley chopped

Directions:

1. Mix everything in a bowl except scallops.
2. Toss in scallops and mix well to coat them.
3. Spread the scallops with the sauce in a baking tray.

4. Press "power button" of air fry oven and turn the dial to select the "bake" mode.
5. Press the Time button and again turn the dial to set the cooking Time to 25 minutes.
6. Now push the temp button and rotate the dial to set the temperature at 350 degrees f.
7. Once preheated, place the scallop's baking tray in the oven and close its lid.
8. Serve warm.

Nutrition: Calories 227 Fat: 10.1g carbohydrate 5.6g protein 27.8g

Crusted Scallops

Preparation Time: 10 minutes

Cooking Time: 20 minutes

Serving: 4

Ingredients:

- `1-1/2 lbs. Bay scallops, rinsed
- `3 garlic cloves, minced
- `1/2 cup panko crumbs
- `1 teaspoon onion powder
- `4 tablespoons butter, melted
- `1/2 teaspoon cayenne pepper
- `1 teaspoon garlic powder
- `1/4 cup parmesan cheese, shredded

Directions:

1. Mix everything in a bowl except scallops.
2. Toss in scallops and mix well to coat them.
3. Spread the scallops with the sauce in a baking tray.
4. Press "power button" of air fry oven and turn the dial to select the "bake" mode.
5. Press the Time button and again turn the dial to set the cooking Time to 20 minutes.

6. Now push the temp button and rotate the dial to set the temperature at 400 degrees f.

7. Once preheated, place the scallop's baking tray in the oven and close its lid.

Nutrition: Calories 242 Fat: 11.1g carbohydrate 11.1g protein 23.8g

Lobster Tails with White Wine Sauce

Preparation Time: 10 minutes

Cooking Time: 14 minutes

Serving: 4

Ingredients:

- `4 lobster tails, shell cut from the top
- `1/2 onion, quartered
- `1/2 cup butter
- `1/3 cup wine
- `1/4 cup honey
- `6 garlic cloves crushed
- `1 tablespoon lemon juice
- `1 teaspoon salt or to taste
- `Cracked pepper to taste
- `Lemon slices to serve
- `2 tablespoons fresh chopped parsley

Directions:

1. Place the lobster tails in the oven's baking tray.
2. Whisk rest of the ingredients in a bowl and pour over the lobster tails.

3. Press "power button" of air fry oven and turn the dial to select the "broil" mode.
4. Press the Time button and again turn the dial to set the cooking Time to 14 minutes.
5. Now push the temp button and rotate the dial to set the temperature at 350 degrees f.
6. Once preheated, place the lobster's baking tray in the oven and close its lid.
7. Serve warm.

Nutrition: Calories 340 Fat: 23.1g carbohydrate 20.4g protein 0.7g

Broiled Lobster Tails

Preparation Time: 10 minutes

Cooking Time: 6 minutes

Serving: 4

Ingredients:

- `2 lobster tails, shell cut from the top
- `1/2 cup butter, melted
- `1/2 teaspoon ground paprika
- `Salt to taste
- `White pepper, to taste
- `1 lemon, juiced

Directions:

1. Place the lobster tails in the oven's baking tray.
2. Whisk rest of the ingredients in a bowl and pour over the lobster tails.
3. Press "power button" of air fry oven and turn the dial to select the "broil" mode.
4. Press the Time button and again turn the dial to set the cooking Time to 6 minutes.
5. Now push the temp button and rotate the dial to set the temperature at 350 degrees f.

6. Once preheated, place the lobster's baking tray in the oven and close its lid.

7. Serve warm.

Nutrition: Calories 227 Fat: 23.1g carbohydrate 0.2g protein 20.3g

Paprika Lobster Tail

Preparation Time: 10 minutes

Cooking Time: 10 minutes

Serving: 4

Ingredients:

- `2 (4 to 6 oz) lobster tails, shell cut from the top
- `1/8 teaspoon salt
- `1/8 teaspoon black pepper
- `1/8 teaspoon paprika
- `2 tablespoon butter
- `1/2 lemon, cut into wedges
- `Chopped parsley for garnish

Directions:

1. Place the lobster tails in the oven's baking tray.
2. Whisk rest of the ingredients in a bowl and pour over the lobster tails.
3. Press "power button" of air fry oven and turn the dial to select the "broil" mode.
4. Press the Time button and again turn the dial to set the cooking Time to 10 minutes.

5. Now push the temp button and rotate the dial to set the temperature at 350 degrees f.

6. Once preheated, place the lobster's baking tray in the oven and close its lid.

7. Serve warm.

Nutrition: Calories 204 Fat: 12.5g carbohydrate 0.2g protein 21.7g

Lobster Tails with Lemon Butter

Preparation Time: 10 minutes

Cooking Time: 8 minutes

Serving: 4

Ingredients:

- `4 lobster tails, shell cut from the top
- `1 tablespoon fresh parsley, chopped
- `2 garlic cloves, pressed
- `1 teaspoon Dijon mustard
- `1/4 teaspoon salt
- `1/8 teaspoon black pepper
- `1-1/2 tablespoon olive oil
- `1-1/2 tablespoon fresh lemon juice
- `4 tablespoon butter, divided

Directions:

1. Place the lobster tails in the oven's baking tray.
2. Whisk rest of the ingredients in a bowl and pour over the lobster tails.
3. Press "power button" of air fry oven and turn the dial to select the "broil" mode.

4. Press the Time button and again turn the dial to set the cooking Time to 8 minutes.
5. Now push the temp button and rotate the dial to set the temperature at 350 degrees f.
6. Once preheated, place the lobster's baking tray in the oven and close its lid.
7. Serve warm.

Nutrition: Calories 281/ fat 18.1g/carbohydrate 0.8g/ protein 27.9g

Sheet Pan Seafood Bake

Preparation Time:10 minutes

Cooking Time: 14 minutes

Serving: 4

Ingredients:

- `2 corn ears, husked and diced
- `1 lb. Red potatoes, boiled, diced
- `2 lbs. Clams, scrubbed
- `1 lb. Shrimp, peeled and de-veined
- `12 oz. Sausage, sliced
- `1/2 red onion, sliced
- `4 lobster tails, peeled
- `Black pepper to taste
- `1 lemon, cut into wedges
- `1 cup butter
- `3 teaspoons minced garlic
- `1 tablespoon old bay seasoning
- `Fresh parsley for garnish

Directions:

1. Toss all the veggies, corn, seafood, oil, and seasoning in a baking tray.

2. Press "power button" of air fry oven and turn the dial to select the "broil" mode.
3. Press the Time button and again turn the dial to set the cooking Time to 14 minutes.
4. Now push the temp button and rotate the dial to set the temperature at 425 degrees f.
5. Once preheated, place the seafood's baking tray in the oven and close its lid.
6. Serve warm.

Nutrition: `Calories 532 Fat: 35.6g carbohydrate 26.3g protein 28.7g

Balsamic Artichokes

Preparation Time:11 minutes

Cooking Time: 8 minutes

Serving: 4

Ingredients:

- 2 tsp of balsamic vinegar
- Black pepper and salt
- 1/4 cup of olive oil
- 1 tsp of oregano
- 4 big trimmed artichokes
- 2 tbsp of lemon juice
- 2 cloves of garlic

Directions:

1. Sprinkle the artichokes with pepper and salt.
2. Brush oil over the artichokes and add lemon juice.
3. Place the artichokes on the Power XL Air Fryer Grill.
4. Set the Power XL Air Fryer Grill at Air fryer/Grill, Timer at 7 minutes at 3600F.
5. Mix garlic, lemon juice, pepper, vinegar, oil in a bowl.

6. Add oregano and salt.

7. Mix well.

8. Serve the artichokes with balsamic vinaigrette.

9. Serving Suggestions: Serve with mint chutney

10. Directions: & Cooking Tips: Use fresh balsamic

Nutrition: Calories: 533kcal, Fat: 29g, Carb: 68g, Proteins: 19g

Cheesy Artichokes

Preparation 15 minutes

Cooking Time:6 minutes

Servings: 5

Ingredients:

- 1 tsp of onion powder
- 1/2 cup of chicken stock
- 14 ounces of artichoke hearts
- 8 ounces of mozzarella
- 1/2 cup of mayonnaise
- 8 ounces of cream cheese
- 10 ounces of spinach
- 3 cloves of garlic
- 16 ounces of grated parmesan cheese
- 1/2 cup of sour cream

Directions:

1. Mix cream cheese, onion powder, chicken stock, and artichokes in a bowl.
2. Add sour cream, mayonnaise, spinach to the bowl.
3. Transfer the mixture to the Power XL Air Fryer Grill pan

4. Set the Power XL Air Fryer Grill to Air fryer/Grill.
5. Set Timer to 6 minutes at 3500F.
6. Serve immediately
7. Serving Suggestions: Serve with parmesan and mozzarella.
8. Directions: & Cooking Tips: Rinse artichokes hearts well.

Nutrition: Calories: 379kcal, Fat: 19g, Carb: 36g, Proteins: 15g

Beet Salad with Parsley Dressing

Preparation Time 15 minutes

Cooking Time:15 minutes

Serving: 4

Ingredients:

- Black pepper and salt
- 1 clove of garlic
- 2 tbsp of balsamic vinegar
- 4 beets
- 2 tbsp of capers
- 1 bunch of chopped parsley
- 1 tbsp of olive oil

Directions:

1. Place bets on the Power XL Air Fryer Grill pan.
2. Set the Power XL Air Fryer Grill to air fry function.
3. Set Timer and temperature to 15 minutes and 3600F.
4. In another bowl, mix pepper, garlic, capers, salt, and olive oil. Mix well

5. Remove the beets from the Power XL Air Fryer Grill and place it on a flat surface.

6. Peel and put it in the salad bowl

7. Serve with vinegar.

8. Serving Suggestions: Dress with parsley mixture.

9. Directions: & Cooking Tips: rinse beets before cooking.

Nutrition: Calories: 185kcal, Fat: 16g, Carb: 11g, Proteins: 8g

Blue Cheese Salad and Beets

Preparation time 15 minutes

Cooking Time:15 minutes

Servings: 5

Ingredients:

- 1 tbsp of olive oil
- Black pepper and salt
- 6 beets
- 1/4 cup of blue cheese

Directions:

1. Set the beets on the Power XL Air Fryer Grill pan.
2. Set the Power XL Air Fryer Grill to air fry function.
3. Set Timer to 15 minutes.
4. Cook at 3500F
5. Transfer it to a plate.
6. Add pepper, blue cheese, oil, and salt.
7. Serve immediately
8. Serving Suggestions: Serve with maple syrup

9. Directions: & Cooking Tips: Peel beets and cut into quarters.

Nutrition: Calories: 110kcal, Fat: 11g, Carb: 4g, Proteins: 5g

Broccoli Salad

Preparation 15 minutes

Cooking Time:9 minutes

Serving: 4

Ingredients:

- 6 cloves of garlic
- 1 head of broccoli
- Black pepper and salt
- 1 tbsp of Chinese rice wine vinegar
- 1 tbsp of peanut oil

Directions:

1. Mix oil, salt, broccoli, and pepper.
2. Place the mixture on the Power XL Air Fryer Grill pan.
3. Set the Power XL Air Fryer Grill to air fry function.
4. Cook for 9 minutes at 3500F.
5. Place the broccoli in the salad bowl and add peanuts oil, rice vinegar, and garlic.
6. Serve immediately.
7. Serving Suggestions: toss the broccoli well in rice vinegar

8. Directions: & Cooking Tips: Separate the broccoli floret

Nutrition: Calories: 199kcal, Fat: 14g, Carb: 17g, Proteins: 8g